# LOCUST BEANS

A nutritional powerhouse

Eliane P. Barrera

Preface

Locust beans is normally processed into food condiment, which is popularly taken in the western part of Africa and it is used as a spice that offers an African meal a first-rate flavor. This paper reviews the roles of locust beans in traditional cuisine and diet, health benefits, culinary uses, traditional and modern recipes, spiritual benefits and common  techniques of manufacturing fermented locust beans, the troubles related with it and the viable approaches of overcoming these issues in order to convey this health friendly seed into the limelight of massive scale production. The processing of locust beans  to meal condiment involves depodding, cleaning, boiling, dehulling, washing, re-cooking and fermentation.

# Contents

- Potential medicinal uses and traditional remedies involving locust beans.

- Culinary uses of locust bean.

- Traditional and modern recipes using locust beans as a key ingredients.

- Method of processing and preparing locust beans for cooking.

- Traditional ways of preserving/sun-drying locust beans.

- The versatility of locust beans spiritually and ritual ceremonies.

## Introduction

Locust beans (Parkia biglobosa) is a multipurpose tree legume positioned in many Africa countries, A dicotyledonous angiosperm belongs to the family fabaceae and is categorized under spermatophytes, vascular plants.

The seeds, the fruit pulp and the leaves are used to put mutual severa foods and drinks and to feed farm animals and poultry.

The African locust bean tree has additionally been observed to possess wonders. For instance, the pulverized bark of the tree is employed in wound healing and serves as one of the ingredients used in treating leprosy. The decoction of the bark is also used as tub for fever and as a warm mouth wash to steam and relieve toothache in Cote d'Ivoire.

Locust beans without a doubt have an influence on controlling blood pressure and the result obtained showed that ample doses of locust beans helped to reduce arterial blood pressure.

The findings showed that the diastolic blood stress dimension enjoyed extra discount than even the systolic blood pressure. It also published the many wonders of the African locust bean tree. The pulverized bark of African locust bean tree, for instance, is employed in wound recuperation and serves as one of the ingredients that are used in treating leprosy.

## An overview of locust beans and historical significance in various cultures

<u>An overview</u>

Locust bean, also known as carob or Saint John's bread, has dark, evergreen, pinnate leaves. The small, pink plant life have no petals. The fruit is a brown, leathery pod about 10–30 cm long and incorporates 10–15 seeds of about 0.2 g each. The seeds are remarkably uniform in measurement and weight.

Parkia biglobosa, popularly known as the "African locust bean tree," has been used in the Nigerian and other West

African rural communities to treat a range of diseases such as malaria, diabetes mellitus, infections, and inflammatory diseases. The efficacy of the quite a number preparations (seeds, leaves, and stem barks) of Parkia biglobosa is widely acclaimed for the remedy of malaria, diabetes mellitus, and painful conditions. The acute toxicity find out about in mice confirmed no lethality and LD50 is higher than 5 g/kg bw, as a result the plant can be a candidate for scientific trial studies.

### Historical significance in various cultures

The tree locust bean (also recognised as "arbre à farine, fern leaf, irú, monkey cutlass tree, two ball nitta-tree, nété and néré") was first written of with the aid of Michael Adamson in 1757's West Africa. The use of fermented locust beans in Africa, however, dates as some distance lower back as the 14th century.

**Scientific name and different regional names of locust beans**

<u>Scientific name</u>

- *Parkia biglobosa*

<u>Different regional names of locust beans</u>

- Dawa dawa/ Iru/Ogiri okpe/Eware in Nigeria
- Afitin/Sonru in Benin
- Soumbala in Burkina Faso
- Netetu in Senegal

**The role of locust beans in traditional cuisines and diets**

- In some societies on the African continent it is no longer an regular meals object but a therapeutic meals and a source of income.

- Locust bean, regularly referred to as iru by way of Yorubas, 'ogiri', 'dawa dawa' via Igbos, is a neighborhood seasoning or condiment used in soups and stews. A very popular soup ingredient, globally, it is referred to as African locust bean with the botanical title as Parkia biglobosa. It is not convenient to seem at, and the smell is disagreeable – at best. These aside, Locust Bean is the single, most full-size ingredient guaranteed to take your soups, stews or blended veggies from just okay to great.

- It can be determined in a wide vary of environments in Africa and is particularly grown for its pods that contain both a sweet pulp and treasured seeds. The most valuable parts of the locust bean are high in lipid (29%), protein (35%), carbohydrate (16%), and is a suitable supply of fats and calcium for rural dwellers. Locust bean product have to be converted into powdery shape and packaged into a range of sizes in plastics for handy distribution.

- Local lookup has proven that locust bean helps to promote excellent sight and drives away hypertension and illnesses conditions like stroke and diabetes. It additionally carries tannins, astringent elements observed in many plants. Foods prosperous in tannins are regularly encouraged for treatment of diarrhea. The element of carob that is made into locust bean gum includes soluble fiber in the galactomannan family. Like different forms of soluble fiber, it has shown workable benefits for enhancing weight loss and controlling blood sugar levels.

- Locust beans are brought to everything – now not only due to the fact it tastes properly and can serve as a tastier choice to other spice cubes, however additionally due to its fitness advantages amongst which are vision improvement, digestion aid and lots more.

Nutritional and anti-nutritional composition of the African locust bean ( Parkia biglobosa ) fruit pulp have been determined using popular methods.

<u>Nutritional composition of locust beans</u>

- A moisture content material of 8.41%,
- Protein 6.56%,
- Fat 1.80%,
- Crude fibre 11.75%,
- Ash. 4.18%
- Carbohydrate of 67.30%.

<u>Sugar content used to be determined</u>

- Complete carotenoids, 49,175ug/ 100g ,
- Ascorbic acid (Vitamin C) of 191.20mg/100g,

- 9° Brix.

<u>Anti-nutritional composition of locust beans</u>

- A phytic acid content of 60.00mg/ 100g; Crude saponins, 17.80mg/ 100g;
- Tannins, 81.00mg/100g;
- Total phenols, 204.60mg/ 100g and Hydrocyanic acid (HCN) content of 17.30mg/ 100g.

**A comprehensive analysis of the nutritional content of locust beans**

Description: Locust Bean, Raw

Local Names: Dorawa (Hausa), Iru (Yoruba), Ogiri okpe (Igbo),

Scientific Name: _Parkia biglobosa_

Category: Condiments and Spices

Calories In Locust Bean

The calories in 100 grams of Locust Bean is 442.46 calories (kcal).


**Macronutrients, Micronutrients, Vitamins and Minerals found in locust beans**


Locust beans macronutrients data

Weight       100g

Energy       1853.655kj

Calories     442.46kcl

Fat.         18.7g

Protein      32.615g

Carb         32.5g

Fiber        6.85g

Water        7.185g


Locust beans mineral data

Weight       100g

Calcium      294.69mg

Iron (Fe)    33.56mg

| Magnesium | 146.18mg |
| Phosphorus (p) | mg |
| Potassium (k) | 932.9mg |
| Sodium (Na) | 107.09mg |
| Zinc (zn) | 27.9mg |
| Copper (cu) | mg |
| Manganese | mg |

<u>Locust beans vitamin data</u>

| Weight | 100g |
| Vit. A, RAE | ug |
| Retinol | mg |
| Carotene, beta | ug |
| Vit. D | ug |
| Thiamine, B1 | mg |
| Riboflavin, B2 | mg |
| Niacin, B3. | mg |
| Vit. B6 | mg |
| Vit. B12 (ug) | ug |
| Folate, B9 (ug) | ug |
| Vit. C (mg) | mg |

<u>Locust beans micronutrients data</u>

Weight          100g

Ash             4.155g

Alcohol         —-

Caffeine        —-

Theobromine  —-

## Comparison of locust beans to other commonly consumed legumes

A large percentage of the world stays in poverty with Nigeria being tagged domestic to the greatest number of the world's poorest. Poverty and malnutrition are two sides of a coin, where poverty exists, hunger follows suit; hungry men and women are chronically undernourished. Poverty is a cause and final result of malnutrition which has a long lasting physiologic effect resulting in a high propensity of fitness challenges at one stage or the other. Thus, low cost source of meals and its derivatives which can meet the nutritional requirement of man will be extensively favored by way of all and sundry. Plant sources may also provide no longer only low-cost and alternative supply of protein, however different nutrients required by man; seeds of P. biglobosa covered as issue of a protein bad weight loss program ought to make up for some of the protein deficiency. Presence of mineral components such as Calcium, Iron, Magnesium, Sodium, Copper, Potassium, Phosphorus, Manganese and Zinc, It is a excellent source of macronutrient, vitamins A and C and carotenoids an desirable level of antinutrient was discovered in a learn about of the_nutritional composition of P. biglobosa where a phytic acid composition of 60.00mg/ 100g was recorded. In a bid to get the excellent out of the seeds, has printed a higher proportion of protein for protein isolate of *P. biglobosa* than the fermented and defatted seeds. It is fascinating to note that the fermented iru does now not accumulate lead and there has been no record of food poisoning in the consumption of fermented *P. biglobosa* bean based totally condiments no matter the detection of cerullude: an emetic toxin producing lines of Bacillus cereus.

Pulp of *P. biglobosa* will make an ideal snack. It has been included into wheat-based biscuits to make functional biscuits and its fruit pulp has been used in the manufacturing of wine. Its fruit hulls are also pronounced to be wealthy in linoleic acid, although its edibility by way of man is to be investigated in contrast to other legumes.

**Health benefits of locust beans**

- It can aid in the cure of diarrhea
- It promotes good eyesight
- Boost fertility
- Healthy muscles
- Treatment of infection
- Remedy of malaria and repellant of mosquito
- Therapy of weight problem and it is ailment complications
- Anti-inflammatory and wound restoration properties
- Treatment of hypertension and manipulation blood pressure

- Treatment of snake bite

- P. biglobosa as a pesticides

- Control of witch weed

- P. biglobosa as an excipient in the pharmaceutical industry

- P. biglobosa as antibacterial and probiotic agent

- P. biglobosa as treatment choice for diabetics

**Exploring the various health benefits associated with consuming locust beans**

- _P. biglobosa_ as antibacterial and probiotic agent

The antibacterial efficacy of P. biglobosa has been validated. Phytochemical screening revealed the presence of alkaloids, flavonoids, tannins, saponins, steroids, glycoside and cardiac glycosides: some of which are responsible for its antibacterial properties. Ethanolic extract of the stem bark of P. biglobosa had a concentration-dependent antimicrobial effect on Pseudomonas aeruginosa, Escherichia coli, Klebsiella pneumoniae, Proteus mirabilis, Aspergillus flavus and Aspergillus fumigatus. The anti-bacterial pastime towards Staphylococcus aureus and Pseudomonas aeruginosa has been demonstrated via investigations.

The antibacterial properties exhibited by means of P. biglobosa may now not only be associated with the constitutive phytochemicals however also to bacteriocin produced through some pressure inherent in the fermented P. biglobosa proven to exhibit probiotic properties. Probiotics are stay organism that confers health advantage on its host when administered in enough amounts. Bacillus subtilis, extensively studied for its probiotic residences and viable incorporation into the manufacturing of novel foods and prophylactic used to be remoted from Soumbala: a fermented product of P. biglobosa. The isolate was proven to inactivate each gram of wonderful and poor micro organisms as nicely as Ochratoxin A producing fungi. In addition, a bacteriocin producing Lactic acid bacteria used to be also isolated from fermented seeds of P. biglobosa

- <u>Treatment of Malaria and repellant of mosquito</u>

Malaria, everyday in malaria endemic regions is transmitted with the aid of the girl anopheles mosquito despite artemisinin-based mixture remedy (ACT) being the quality capsules for its treatment, flora nonetheless remain the key source for antimalarial. P. biglobosa as one of the most referred to plant used in the remedy of malaria. The stem bark decoction and smoke of the seed pills is used to treat malaria and as a mosquito repellant respectively.

- <u>Treatment of weight problem and it is ailment complications</u>

Body mass index (BMI) is broadly speaking used to categorize underweight, normal, overweight and obese individuals. Worldwide, the incidence of Obesity is expected to grow by 40%. Obesity is a threat issue implicated without delay and indirectly as a cause of the continual as nicely as the degenerative forms of ailments of the kidney, liver and heart.

The propensity for overweight character to go through from a range of disorder that should be terminal triggered the search no longer only for high quality measures to shed weight however for capability_of treating and possibly curing the ailments associated with it.

Change in life-style through food plan and weight loss therapy is a most guaranteed skill of managing weight problems and its related complications. A decoction of the root or stem of P. biglobosa is used for weight loss remedies. In the equal study, the bark and seeds had been stated to have potentials in urge for food suppression. These normal claims want to be scientifically analyzed to produce novel plant based totally products for weight loss reduction.

Disease effects of weight problems from kidney, liver and heart may want to be managed and handled via P.

biglobosa; this is demonstrated the place its leaves were purportedly used in treating kidney disorders. The undertaking of P. biglobosa is stated to be same with Acetylycysteine: a trendy reference hepatoprotective drug, in decreasing serum Alkaline Phosphatase and Aspartate with a non-significant effect on Alkaline phosphatase when the methanolic extract of its stem bark was used to assay its hepatoprotective impact on paracetamol cause liver damage in wistar rats. It is mentioned to be in a position to maintain liver features and protective against CCl4 triggered liver damage in combination with Negro pepper -Xylopia ethiptica.

- _P. biglobosa_ as treatment choice for diabetics

About 3.1 million humans with Diabetics in Nigeria, an international dying toll of 3.8 million is recorded annually. This disorder is characterized through high sugar ranges in the blood and in spite of its administration clinically, death occurs. Oral

Hypoglycemic therapy, Insulin treatment and dietary modifications are the main thing of treating Diabetics.

A keystone in obtaining a suitable glycemic manage in DM patients can be completed by way of modification in diet.

Butanolic fraction of leaves of *P. biglobosa* has been used to stimulate β cells function, result in insulin manufacturing with a corresponding discount in blood sugar degree and also decrease different complications related with Type 2 DM when administered to Type 2 DM triggered rats. Aqueous and Ethanolic extract of fermented P. biglobosa seeds was once additionally proven to possess antidiabetic homes with the aqueous extract restoring weight misplaced associated with DM.

Lupeol a triterpene was once remoted from P. biglobosa. This compound and some of its ester derivatives whose main mechanism of motion is inhibition of the enzyme α amylase, has been proven to possess antidiabetic prowess.

- <u>Anti-inflammatory and wound restoration homes</u>

Inflammatory mediators released from broken tissues stimulate nociceptors at once and this may also relief pain,

However this constitutes a section of the wound recuperation process. Inflammatory ache is dealt with by way of nonsteroidal anti inflammatory pills and coxibs however their use are related with damaging effects.

Antinociceptive exercise related to the inhibition of inflammatory methods is exhibited by using lectin isolated from Parkia biglobosa.

The ground bark of this plant is used to make decoction for treating various forms of wound and for making paste for wound dressing. The success portrayed with the aid of common healers may be the capability of Parkia biglobosa to stimulate the increase of fibroblast. Fibroblast is responsible for collagen and elastin synthesis which is important in the wound healing process, It is key in wound contraction where it gives the contractile pressure that brings the wound edges together. Asthma, a lower respiratory disorder affecting all ages, is characterized by using a continual airway infection culminating in the narrowing of the airway. The financial cost on patients is substantial and Its administration contributes to societal fitness care cost. Inhaled corticosteroid are by and large believed through physicians as the benchmark for the administration of asthma but its use is attributed to some crucial side-effects which has brought on some patient to discontinue treatment and to the poor response of corticosteroid resistant asthma sufferers to its administration, consequently requiring higher dosage. In a survey carried out 85.7% of medical practitioners and 56.0% of sufferers agreed on the need for new medicine choices that are greater effective; this demand is also documented.

Alternative plant based therapy of allergies can also be less costly compared to the conventional scientific management.

*Parkia biglobosa* has been used via Togolese regular healers to heal asthma. Other works such as additionally cited its use in treating asthma.

- *P. biglobosa* as an excipient in the pharmaceutical industry

Inert pharmaceutical elements used in product formulations called excipients could serve a specific purpose which may want to be: binder or adhesives, disintegrant, lubricants, glidant, flavors, colors and sweeteners and pH adjustment. A binder imparts cohesiveness and ensures a tablet stays intact after compression. The pulps of *P.biglobosa* has high water sorption efficiency which should be incorporated into the pharmaceutical industry, it additionally has potentials in being used as a binder and thickener.

- Control of witch weed

Striga gesnerioides (witch weed) is a parasitic weed that constrains the productivity of staple crops; entire crop loss ought to be skilled in Striga infestation which may also continue to be doable in the soil for up to 20 years (AATF, 2012). A variety of administration techniques has been proffered through the scientific neighborhood with crop rotation topping the list, others encompass intercropping with Striga host and non☐host crops, elevated fallow and soil fertility management, biological control. Innovative management system that pursue the eradication of witch weed will increase the productiveness of staple crops. The fruit powder of P. biglobosa reduced the range of Striga gesnerioides in cowpea cropping device with the basal software of the fruit pulp recording a greater grain yield and decreasing Striga count.

- <u>P. biglobosa as a pesticide</u>

Dimethoate is an organophosphate acaricide that inhibits the enzyme cholinesterase responsible for lysing various ester primarily based choline neurotransmitters in the apprehensive and cardiovascular system, lungs, plasma, red blood cell, skin and eyes. Dimethoate synergizes with Cypermethrin: a regarded neurotoxic category II pyrethroid pesticide.

Aqueous, pod husk extract of P. biglobosa is comparable to plants handled with 2.5ml of the insecticide Dimethoate Cypermethrin when its capacity to suppress flea beetles in okro manufacturing used to be investigated.

- <u>Treatment of snake bite</u>

Several flora are used both as a first useful resource to snake chunks or as an everlasting cure. Pharmacological basis of some of these flowers can also not have been established, this has however no longer stopped their usage. The efficiency of the methanolic extract of P. biglobosa stem bark against the cytotoxic, haemotoxic and neurotoxic, and consequences of venoms of venomous snakes has been confirmed in a study.

- <u>It promotes good eyesight</u>

Locust beans make imaginative and prescient clearer, their consumption helps_to give desirable eyesight to human beings who have eye issues such as cataract, minus eyes, myopia, glaucoma and the rest due to the fact they also contain herbal nutrients that can keep eye health.

Beans and legumes (such as chickpeas, black-eyed peas, kidney beans, and lentils) are a first-rate food alternative for eye health. They are vegetarian, low-fat, and excessive in fiber and zinc, and the nutrients they contain help shield the retina and lower your hazard for creating cataracts.

It is one of the actual sources of protein, Vitamin A, Sodium, Iron, Zinc, Calcium and Potassium.

- <u>It can aid in the cure of diarrhea</u>

Locust beans can serve as a local remedy for diarrhea, (which is a circumstance where a person excretes in liquid structure repeatedly) because it consists of a nutrient referred to as tannis and the substance works for diarrhea remedy, Because of the quantity of tannin determined in African locust bean, it will heal diarrhea, which is a gastrointestinal disease with the signs of common watery bowel movements. Consuming African locust beans will assist you relieve diarrhea

- ### Treatment of hypertension and manipulation blood pressure

African locust bean has been put on research and examined to locate the effects and it is proven that it can manipulate blood pressure because it helps in lowering arterial blood strain when you consume the right.

Hypertension, a blood pressure level that is $\geq$ 140mmHg or 90mmHg in the systole and diastole respectively doubles the incidence of cardiovascular chance in an character American Diabetes Association (2008) It's regularly now not detected and when diagnosed, often not appropriately handled accordingly there is a need to stop this silent killer.

A variety of literatures such as have attested to the antihypertensive houses of *P. biglobosa*. The Bogou team of Togo who fed on a excessive amount of the fermented seeds confirmed a extensive decrease in blood stress and heart beat in contrast to the a crew who do now not eat it at all: the Goumou-kope area, when Investigations into the antihypertensive prowess of *P. biglobosa* thru anthropometric, medical and biochemical analyses have been carried out in Togo also printed that seeds of P. biglobosa immediately acted on smooth muscle by the endothelium to generate vasodilating prostaglandins in rat aorta, it is cited in an ethnobotanical survey through as one of the most frequently used plant in treating hypertension by Togoleses typical healer.

- <u>Locust beans boost fertility</u>

Locust beans include zinc which, in accordance to research, will increase testosterone levels. Research has additionally shown that this mineral can enhance the potency and frequency of sexual intercourse.

Another reason you need to add locusts beans to your weight-reduction plan is to raise your immune system. Locust beans comprise zinc, a hint issue that makes you less inclined to disease and illness.

Fiber and folate help the body hold healthy hormone balances and lentils, in precise incorporation of high levels of the polyamine spermidine, which may help sperm fertilize the egg. Include chickpeas, cannellini beans or black beans, and add yellow lentils, red lentils or black lentils to stews or soups.

- <u>Treatment of infection</u>

*Parkia biglobosa*, popularly known as the "African locust bean tree," has been used in the Nigerian and other West African rural communities to deal with a variety of illnesses such as malaria, diabetes mellitus, infections, and inflammatory diseases . The efficacy of a variety of preparations (seeds, leaves, and stem barks) of *Parkia biglobosa* is widely acclaimed for the treatment of malaria, diabetes mellitus, and painful conditions. The acute toxicity study in mice confirmed no lethality and LD50 is increased to 5 g/kg bw, hence the plant can be a candidate for clinical trial studies.

African locust beans have been used historically in Nigeria and different West African rural communities to deal with a range of diseases along with ulcer associated diseases. Methanol extracts and fractions from the stem bark of African locust bean tree were evaluated for their anti-ulcer activity using ethanol and acetyl salicylic acid (ASA) as the ulcerogens. The extract and fraction have been administered orally at the doses of 100, 200 and 400 mg/kg b. wt. for the experimental businesses whilst the manage and reference corporations acquired distilled water (2 ml/kg, p.o) and omeprazole (20 mg/kg, p.o) respectively. The oral median deadly dose LD50 in mice used to be estimated to be increased than 5000 mg/kg and the phytochemical analysis revealed the presence of anthraquinones, flavonoids, phenols, saponins, steroids, tannins, and terpenes while flavonoids, tannins and terpenes have been current in the fraction.

The effects show that the extract and fraction drastically (p < 0.05) reduced the ulcer index from 13 ± 1.25 to three ± 0.99, 13 ± 1.25 to 5.20 ± 0.31 and from 12.0 ± 0.68 to 2.81 ± 0.79, 12.0 ± 0.68 to 4.40± 0.67 in the ethanol and ASA triggered ulceration respectively. Percentage ulcer inhibitions of extract and fraction at 400 mg/kg for ethanol and ASA triggered ulcers have been 79.9, 60.0, 76.7 and 63.3 p.c respectively. African locust bean tree stem bark is a practicable supply of a new anti-ulcer agent.

- <u>Healthy muscles</u>

Rich in Amino Acids: Locust beans are an exact supply of vital amino acids, which are the building blocks of proteins. These amino acids are essential for a number of bodily functions, consisting of muscle growth, immune machine support, and tissue repair.

The protein and amino acids composition of seeds and pulp of African locust beans (*Parkia biglobosa*) had been analyzed. The protein content material (in % dry matter) of seeds with and without hull used to be determined to be 28.20% and 32.40% respectively while that of pulp is 1.84%. The results for amino acids evaluation point out that the seeds are the true source of most quintessential amino acids in which each complete and dehulled seed has a chemical rating of 5/8 together with the sulfur-containing amino acids. Pulp has a chemical rating of 1/8. Threonine and lysine are the most limiting indispensable amino acids in seeds and pulp respectively. These consequences should serve as a database for encouraging the normal population in particular the masses in growing international locations to harness the nutritional manageability of wildly happening plant meals for narrowing nutritional deficiencies.

**The role of locust beans in promoting heart health, food digestion and absorption and immunity.**

- <u>Heart health</u>

Cardiovascular Health: Locust beans' mixture of fiber, potassium, and antioxidants supports cardiovascular fitness via promoting healthful blood strain and reducing the risk of heart disease.

- <u>Food digestion and absorption</u>

Lipids in your body are indispensable for desirable digestion and absorption of food and nutrients. These lipids can be determined in locust beans, and are wished to transport fat-soluble vitamins—A, D, E and K from the intestines to the bloodstream to make certain absorption of food nutrients.

Besides aiding in everyday bowel movements, the fiber in locust beans can support a healthy gut microbiome. A balanced intestine microbiome is associated with accelerated digestion and usual well-being.

- <u>Immunity</u>

Immune System Support: The nutritional vitamins and minerals discovered in locust beans, such as vitamin C, iron, and zinc, play a role in assisting a wholesome immune system. A sturdy immune machine helps the body shield against infections and illnesses.

 Antioxidant Power: Locust beans are packed with antioxidants, consisting of vitamin C and flavonoids. Antioxidants assist guard the body from oxidative stress and free radicals, doubtlessly decreasing the danger of chronic diseases.

**Potential medicinal uses and traditional remedies involving locust beans**

<u>Traditional medicinal uses</u>

Parkia species are being used across all tropical international locations to remedy unique ailments. Virtually, all components of Parkia plants are utilized historically for special medicinal purposes. The materials of one of a kind parts of Parkia plants are processed as paste, decoction, and juice for the remedy of a range of ailments. Almost all reported Parkia species are used in distinct forms to remedy diarrhea and dysentery.

Different parts of *P. biglobosa, P. clappertoniana, P. roxburghii, and P. speciosa* are reported to be traditionally used for the cure of diabetes.

Furthermore, skin-related diseases, such as eczema, skin ulcers, measles, leprosy, wound, dermatitis, chickenpox, scabies, and ringworm are handled the use of leaves, pods, and roots of *P. speciosa and P. timoriana.*

The stem barks of *P. bicolor, P. clappertoniana, P. biglobosa, P. roxburghii* as properly as roots of *P. speciosa* are utilized in the structure of paste and decoction to treat one of a kind skin problems]. Decoction and paste of stem bark, pod, or root of P. biglobosa and P. speciosa are used to treat hypertension.

Moreover, stem barks of *P. bicolor, P. biglobosa* and leaves of *P. speciosa* are used for extreme cough and bronchitis. These aforementioned makes use of counseled that Parkia plants are probably to include materials with vast and various biological activities, such as antidiabetic, antimicrobial, antihypertensive, and anti-inflammatory.

- <u>Antimicrobial Activity</u>

Various parts of many species of *Parkia* have good antimicrobial activities. They are most active against *S. aureus* and *E. coli.* So far, there is nevertheless no scientific learn about carried out on the plant life investigating the activity. Enormous reports have been made on antimicrobial undertakings of exclusive parts of P. biglobosa such as stem bark, root and pod. Furthermore, the stem barks and leaves of P. clappertoniana aqueous and methanol extracts investigated on some Gram-positive and Gram-negative microorganisms published that both stem barks and leaves have been wonderful in all examined organisms, but methanol extract was more potent. The ethanol extract of both leaves and barks established growth inhibitory effects on multi-drug resistant Salmonella and Shigella isolates. The ethanol extract of P. platycephala seeds tested against six microorganism traces and three yeasts showed no antimicrobial activity. However, lectin acquired from the seed used to be mentioned to notably beautify antibiotic endeavor of gentamicin against S. aureus and E. coli multi-resistant traces due to interaction between carbohydrate-binding website of the lectin and the antibiotic.

In *P. speciosa*, the water suspension of the seeds shows some excellent inhibitory activity against bacteria remoted from the moribund fishes and shrimps—S. aureus, A. hydrophila, S. agalactiae, *S. anginosus and V. parahaemolyticus*—but no detectable activity against *E. coli, V. alginolyticus, E. tarda, C. freundii, and V. vulnificus*. The methanol, chloroform, and petroleum ether extracts of the seeds reveal boom inhibitory effect against H. pylori, whilst the ethyl acetate extract against E. coli, but no effect on S. typhi, S. sonnei, and S. typhimurium. The antimicrobial endeavor of P. speciosa is attributable to the presence of cyclic polysulfides 85 and 92–94 in the seeds. However, the feasible mechanism of the polysulfides was once no longer elucidated. Both pod extract and its synthesized silver nanoparticles exhibit antibacterial activity, with the latter suggesting higher pastime against P. aeruginosa [. A comparable antibacterial endeavor is additionally viewed with aqueous extract of P. speciosa leaves and its silver nanoparticles against *S. aureus, B. subtilis, E. coli, and P. aeruginosa.*

Its bark methanol extract inhibits the increase of Gloeophyllum trabeum, however not Pycnoporus sanguineus, whose impact is no longer seen with each sapwood and heartwood of the plant. Its ethyl acetate extract of the peel additionally shows four instances greater pastime against S. aureus and three instances higher against E. coli than streptomycin, but n-hexane extract exhibits decreased activity.

Various components of P. timoriana inhibit the increase of *B. cereus, V. cholerae, E. coli,* and *S. aureus.* Its leaf extract reveals giant growth inhibitory impact against E. coli, V. cholerae, S. aureus, and B. cereus, whilst its gold and silver nanoparticles from dried leaves inhibit S.

aureus growth. The recreation is believed to be attributable to the accumulation and absorption of the gold and silver nanoparticles into S. aureus cell wall. The methanol extract and semi-polar fractions (chloroform and ethyl acetate) of the bark show significant inhibitory consequences against Neisseria gonorrhoeae. The chloroform extract suggests nice activity. The aqueous extract of the seed, leaf and skin pod also possess antimicrobial activity.

Acetone, ethanol and aqueous extracts of P. biglandulosa stem bark have been among the plant extracts that show the very best antimicrobial endeavor against microorganism and fungi as well as plant pathogenic bacteria. The methanol extract of the leaves also suggests excellent growth inhibition against *E. coli, P. aeruginosa, and S. aureus*. Investigation on *P. bicolor* indicates that ethyl acetate, ethanol, and aqueous extracts of the leaves display a concentration-dependent increase inhibitory effect in opposition to some Gram-positive of bacteria such as *E. coli, S. aureus, P. aeruginosa, A. niger, B. cereus, and a fungus, C. utilis*. Methanol, ethyl acetate, and water extracts of the root additionally show off unique degrees of inhibition towards some frequent human pathogenic bacteria including C. *diphtheriae, K. pneumoniae, P. mirabilis, S. typhi, and S. pyogenes.* The feasible mechanism of the antimicrobial recreation of Parkia plants are but to be determined. However, terpenoids from the vegetation could result in lipid flippase recreation in the bacterial cellular membrane which then enhances membrane injury for a higher phone penetration. Other feasible actions should be by way of damaging bacterial protein, inhibiting DNA gyrase and DNA synthesis, which are but to be validated in further studies.

Collectively, it can be concluded that the antimicrobial homes of Parkia plants rely on the species and components of Parkia as properly as solvent (polar and nonpolar). Most of the published documents are in vitro evaluations, which do not guarantee the same consequences in animal fashions and scientific settings. In the rise of resistant pathogenic bacteria to antimicrobial therapy, there is a pressing need to increase new antimicrobial agents, and phytoconstituents from plants like Parkia could be excellent candidates.

- <u>Antidiabetic Activity</u>

*P. speciosa* is the most studied among different species for antidiabetic activity. Six studies comprising three in vitro and three in vivo studies have established hypoglycemic recreation of the plant, but no medical study has been conducted. Most of the research has studied the endeavor in the seeds and pods.

Pericarps from *P. speciosa* show tremendous inhibitory exercise (IC50 0.0581 mg/mL; 89.46%) towards α-glucosidase, an enzyme responsible for breaking down starch and polysaccharide into glucose. The seeds additionally exhibit inhibitory undertaking however at a lower percentage (45.72%). In every other study, the ethanol extract of the rind had the very best α-glucosidase inhibitory endeavor followed by means of the leaf and seed with IC50 of 4596 ppm, 54,341 ppm, and 67,425 ppm, respectively as compared with acarbose having 162,508 ppm.

An in vivo study conducted on each seeds and pods of P. speciosa in alloxan-induced diabetic rats, indicated that solely chloroform extract of each pods and seeds exhibited robust glucose-lowering activity. The hypoglycemic activity of the seeds was greater than that of the pods (57% and 36%, respectively). A combination of 66% $\beta$-sitosterol 60 and 34% stigmasterol 61 is believed to be responsible for the hypoglycemic impact of the seeds—demonstrated 83% decrease in blood glucose level (100 mg/kg body weight) compared to glibenclamide (111% at five mg/kg bw). Similarly, stigmast-4-en-3-one 63 was identified as the compound responsible for the 84% discount in blood glucose level at one hundred mg/kg bw of the pod extract of P. speciosa. Both compounds ($\beta$-sitosterol and stigmasterol) are believed to minimize blood glucose degree through regenerating remnant $\beta$-cells and stimulating insulin release via augmentation of GLUT4 glucose transporter expression. Stigmasterol is also mentioned to inhibit the ß-cells apoptosis.

In other *Parkia* species, methanol crude extracts and fractions of P. timoriana pods confirmed widespread α-glucosidase and α-amylase inhibitory activities in streptozotocin-induced diabetic rats. Ethyl acetate fraction had the absolute best α-glucosidase inhibitory and average α-amylase inhibitory activities, with maximal discount in blood glucose level again to everyday observed on day 14 at the dose of 100 mg/kg physique weight . α-Amylase features to hydrolyze starch into maltose and glucose. Bioassay-guided chemical investigation of the most energetic ethyl acetate fraction printed epigallocatechin gallate 4 and apigenin 14 were accountable for the antidiabetic activity.

Oral administration of *P. biglobosa* methanol and aqueous extracts of fermented seeds exhibited unique levels of hypoglycemic effects on fasting plasma glucose when tested on alloxan-induced diabetic rats after 4 weeks. Oral administration of *a* seeds methanol extract

(1 g/kg body weight) reduced blood glucose by way of 44.1% at 8 h as compared with glibenclamide (37.9%) in alloxan-induced diabetic rats. Its chloroform fraction exerted the most glucose-lowering impact (65.7%), whilst n-hexane fraction had the lowest (4.7%). As in the past mentioned, a comparable underlying mechanism of the hypoglycemic pastime of the plant species is counseled which is with the aid of an enhancement in pancreatic islet features to launch insulin, while abolishing insulin resistance.

- <u>Anticancer Activity</u>

Cancer is one of the ailments that motive loss of life of millions worldwide. Dietary consumption of uncooked seeds was once also suggested to drastically decrease the occurrence of esophageal most cancers in southern Thailand. The methanol extract of P. speciosa seeds exhibited a moderate antimutagenic pastime in the Ames test, but vulnerable pastime in Epstein–Barr virus inhibitory assay. The methanol extract of the seed coats proven selective cytotoxicity against MCG-7 and T47D (breast cancer), HCT-116 (colon cancer) and HepG2 (hepatocarcinoma) cells, while its ethyl acetate fraction only showed selective cytotoxicity against MCF-7, breast cancer cells.

Substances that beautify mitogenesis of lymphocytes might also be useful as antitumor or antiproliferative and immunomodulator agents. Lectin acquired from the P. speciosa seeds exerted mitogenic exercise in each rat thymocytes and human lymphocytes via stimulating the incorporation of thymidine into DNA cell, which exercise was once related to the recognized T-cell mitogens like pokeweed mitogen, concanavalin A and phytohemagglutinin. Lectins removed from the seeds of P. biglandulosa and P. roxburghii have verified antiproliferative impact on murine macrophage, most cancers mobile phone lines—P 388 DI and J774. The seed extract P. roxburghii also inhibits the proliferation of B-cell hybridoma mobile phone line, HB98, and HepG2 cells except affecting the normal cells. The monosaccharide saponins 52–55 isolated from P. bicolor root also showcase reasonable antiproliferative impact

IC50 ranging from 48.49 to 81.66 µM. To our knowledge, the anticancer outcomes of *Parkia* extracts had been solely investigated in mobile phone lines—limited to telephone growth inhibition—not but studied in in vivo models.

An in vitro find out about on human most cancers cell phone traces has shown that the methanol extracts of P. biglobosa and P. filicoides exhibit special ranges of antiproliferative activities on T-549 and BT-20 (prostate cancer), PC-3 (acute T cell leukemia Jurka), and SW-480 (colon cancer) at concentrations of 20 and two hundred µg/mL. P. biglobosa also reveals higher cytotoxic activity in opposition to all types of most cancers mobile phone strains used compared with P. filicoides. The antitumor property may want to be attributable to the antiangiogenic undertaking of some species of Parkia such as P. biglandulosa and P. speciosa extracts. Angiogenesis or neovascularization is worried in metastasis of strong tumors. Methanol extract of the P. speciosa fresh pods was reported to exhibit antiangiogenic pastime by using more than 50%

inhibition of microvessel outgrowth in rat aortae and human umbilical vein endothelial cells forming capillary-like constructions in Matrigel matrix. The impact might also be attributable to the ability of the compounds in the extract to form vacuoles in the cells, which is vital in keeping the viability of the cells, consequently advisable in the therapy of most cancers owing to its capacity to stop tumor neovascularization.

The plant bioactive compounds may want to additionally maybe extend apoptotic signaling pathway with the aid of elevating caspase activation as similarly shown by using the identical compounds in other plant species, as nicely as a direct inhibition on DNA synthesis, related to the capability to inhibit the expressions of countless tumor- and angiogenesis-associated genes. Future studies ought to explore the viable mechanisms of motion that are responsible for the anticancer activity.

- <u>Antianemic Activity</u>

The fermented seeds of P. biglobosa are a rich supply of critical minerals such as iron, calcium, thiamine, and phosphorus which are vital in forestalling either iron or non-iron deficiency anemia. Therefore, the antianemic capacity of P. biglobosa could be owing to its dietary composition. The fermented seeds of P. biglobosa in aggregate with other fermented products had been said to be beneficial in the administration of anemia as it extended hemoglobin, purple blood cells, white blood cells, and packed telephone volume. The ethanol extract of P. speciosa seeds had been also investigated in NaNO2-induced anemic mice. At doses of 400 and seven-hundred mg/kg, an elevation of hemoglobin ranges used to be noted to 0.92 and 0.82 g/dL, respectively. The specific mechanism of how P. speciosa acts to minimize anemia is nonetheless unclear. It should be due to its rich supply of the minerals, particularly the iron. Another feasible mechanism_would be stimulation of the erythropoiesis process. Both extracts of P. biglobosa P. biglobosa and P. speciosa can be developed as a choice iron supplement. However, the effectiveness can be evaluated clinically.

Daily consumption of cooked pods of P. roxburghii does no longer impose any sizable negative effect. However, consuming raw pods may additionally end up resulting in horrific breath owing to its wealthy content in unstable disulfide compounds, which are exhaled in breath and the scent can persist for a range of hours. Many elements have been identified or removed from Parkia seed, such as lectins, non-protein amino acids, and alkaloids. However, no acute mortality and observable behavioral exchange have been recorded at doses up to 2000 mg/kg ethyl acetate fraction of P. roxburghii pod in rats. Investigation on acute and sub-acute toxicity profiles of the aqueous and ethanol extracts of the stem bark of P. biglobosa showed that the oral median lethal dose (LD50) was once as soon as greater than 5000 mg/kg for every extract in rats. However, in every other report, LD50 values of the leaves, stems and roots in an acute toxicity discovered out abouthad been within the vary of 500–5000 mg/kg physique weight of fish, suggesting that they are solely barely poisonous and, therefore, no longer probable dangerous. The detrimental results blanketed respiratory misery and agitated behavior. Apart from the barks of P. biglobosa, the pods moreover possess the piscicidal venture that can be used in the administration and manipulation of fishponds to get rid of predators. Fatty acids and oils identified from the seeds of P. biglobosa and P. bicolor were said to be non-toxic.

The aqueous extract of P. clappertoniana seeds confirmed no observable maternal and developmental toxicity at 100–500 mg/kg when given orally to Sprague-Dawley rats and mice at particular gestational age.  P. platycephala leaves at a thousand mg/kg on the unique hand, added about decreases in physique mass, meals and water consumption in rats. It additionally shortened the proestrus and extended diestrus phases, as right as lowered uterine weight, suggestive of viable differences on hormonal levels, but no apparent toxicity on different organs. Oral administration of the leaves of P. speciosa for 14 days showed no substantial histopathological toxicity or mortality in rats at up to

5000 mg/kg. In vitro, the plant pods (100 µg/mL) verified no significant cytotoxicity have an impact on normal cell phone lines. Consumption of the seeds up to 30 portions in a serve does now not produce any dangerous results.

## Culinary uses of locust beans

It is used for local seasoning of soups, from bitter-leaf soup, okra soup to fried pepper stew for local rice. Indeed, the fermented seeds of Parkia biglobosa or African locust bean tree are used in all components of Nigeria and the West Coast of Africa for seasoning regular soups.

African locust beans when boiled and fermented are rich in lipid (29 %), protein (35 %), carbohydrate (16 %) quintessential vitamins and minerals such as calcium, fat, potassium, Vitamin C and phosphorus.

Processing locust bean seeds is very indispensable as it helps to boost its dietary value, reduces its natural or artificial compounds that avoid the absorption of nutrients, boosts its digestibility and enriches its unique flavor in order to raise the smell and style of food.

If you are new to locust beans, right here are some ways to comprise them into your diet:

Soup Seasoning: Use locust beans as a herbal seasoning in your soups and stews. They impart an awesome flavor.

Sauces and Gravies: Add ground locust beans to your sauces and gravies for a special taste.

Stir-Fries: Sprinkle locust beans over your vegetable stir-fries for a contact of smokiness.

Marinades: Mix crushed locust beans with spices and herbs to create a flavorful marinade for meats or vegetables.

Dips and Spreads: Blend locust beans with components like garlic, olive oil, and lemon juice to make a scrumptious dip or spread.

**Traditional and modern recipes using locust beans as a key ingredients**

- <u>Locust beans seasoning</u>

Ingredients

Locust beans

Ginger

Dried pepper

Black pepper

Crayfish

Clove

Cooking Instructions

Step 1

Dry your locust beans and set side

Step 2

In a pan toast your other supplies apart from crayfish and allow to cool.

Step 3

Add all of the substances to your blender and blend till smooth, change to a tight container and use later.

- <u>Locust beans rice</u>

Ingredients

4 cups rice

Palm oil

Cumin powder

Garlic powder

Cinnamon powder

Maggi

Salt

Locust beans

Dry fish

Beef

Dry pepper

Onions

Cooking Instructions

Step 1

Parboil your rice

Note: I used the everyday Nigerian close by rice, so you can use any rice of your preference (basmati,foreign or brown rice)

Step 2

In a pot,heat your oil and add in the diced onions and permit it fry for few minutes

Add in your cumin,garlic and cinnamon powder, stir it

Step 3

Add in your locust beans,dry fish and beef

Step 4

Add water and your rice then permit it to cook

Step 5

Enjoy your food

- <u>Locust bean jollof pasta</u>

Ingredients

Cooking duration: 30 mins

2 sachet pasta(spaghetti)

Palm Oil

Grounded Locust beans(daddawa)

Onion

Scallion

Carrot

Grated tata sai and chili

cloves Fresh garlic

Seasoning

Pepper flakes

Dried-powdered ginger

Cooking Instructions

Step 1

Blanch pasta and set aside

Step 2

In a smooth dry pan, pour in palm oil and fry onion

Step 3

Then grated chili/tatasai

Step 4

Chopped carrots

Step 5

G. Locust beans

Step 6

Scallion

Step 7

Seasoning/spices and stir-fry for 3mins

Step 8

In a huge pan, pour in spaghetti

Step 9

Then sauce

Step 10

Keep stirring till well combined

Step 11

And here it is ready


<u>Spaghetti with locust bean(dawadawa)</u>

Ingredients

Golden penny spaghetti

Locust bean powder (garin dawadawa)

Salt,Maggi, and onga

Veg oil

Blended tattasai,attarugu, ginger & fresh garlic

Sliced onions

Cooking Instructions

Step 1

In a neat pot and veg,oil,your blended items stir fry add onions and dawadawa fry for few seconds add water to the same amount of your spaghetti when the water boil add the spaghetti and seasoning reduce the fire to cook slowly and give out a nice taste,now your locust beans spaghetti is ready!

<u>Nigeria white rice, beans and locust beans</u>

Ingredients

Nigerian Rice

White beans

Pepper (roughly ground)

Shambu (roughly ground)

Iru (fresh locust beans)

Spring onions (sliced)

Palm oil

Salt

Maggi seasoning

Lettuce

Cucumber

Boiled eggs

Cooking Instructions

Step 1

Put water in pot on fire, onces it boils, wash rice entirely easy and add to the pot with salt, stir and cover to cook (soft)

Step 2

In any other small pot of water on fire, wash smooth beans and add to the water with little salt cowl to cook dinner well

Step 3

Put pot on fire, add palm oil enable to heat, add spring onions stir, add pepper and shambu stir well till shallow fry

Step 4

Add easy locust beans to the fried substances stir, add salt with seasoning and little water, cover for some minutes

Step 5

Wash proper lettuce to do away with dirts and chop the usage of knife

Step 6

Clean cucumber and cut into spherical slice and cubes

Step 7

Dice the boiled eggs

Step 8

Dish out the cooked rice, beans, sauce and garnish with lettuce

Step 9

Serve hot with a drink of desire.

<u>Locust bean jellof rice</u>

Ingredients

Palm oil

Blended, peppers and onions

Chopped spring onions

Smoked fish

Diced carrots

Seasoning

Locust beans powder

Ginger powder

Garlic powder

Rice

Cooking Instructions

Step 1

Fry the palm oil with some onions. Add in the pepper mix and the smoked fish and fry.

Step 2

Add in water, all the powders, enough locust beans and seasoning.

Step 3

Allow to cook now, not simply boil. Add in washed rice. After it is almost cooked, add in the sliced carrots and spring onions. Put the flame to the lowest and allow it to steam.

Step 4

Ready to serve.

<u>Simple palm oil jellof rice and beans with locust beans</u>

Ingredients

11 cups rice

2 cup beans

1 cup palm oil

1 teaspoon locust beans powder

4 seasoning cubes

1/2 desk spoon salt

1 large rice spoonful of combo peppers

2 large onions (Sliced)

Cooking Instructions

Step 1

Wash the beans and add two cups of water, Sliced onions
in it to help cook it faster, boil for 30 mins or less
depending on the kind of beans and how tender it is.

Step 2

In a separate pot, fry the red oil with onions, add in the
blended pepper, onions and locust beans, fry for two

mins, then add two cups of water to the contents of the pot, add the seasonings and salt, let it boil.

Step 3

Add the boiled beans, wash the rice and add, stir and close the pot, let it prepare dinner for 30_40 mins, or until the water dries up and rice is soft, you can slice in onions on top and close the pot to let it steam for 5mins.

<u>Traditional jellof rice with locust beans</u>

Ingredients

2 cups of rice

½ vegetable oil

1 large onions

Blended pepper and crayfish

2 Maggi cubes

Seasoning

Locust beans

Little salt

Step 1

Get a clean pot put on warmness pour water and pour your rice parboil for 8 minutes after which you wash the rice with a filter put back the clean pot on warmth

Step 2

Pour your vegetable oil in the pot enable to hot then you add your blended pepper and onion and additionally your blended crayfish stir fry for 2 minutes thereafter you add a cup of water cowl the pot and allow it to boil after which you add your maggi cubes, a pinch of salt and the locust beans cover the pot so that the ingredients can combine excellent

Step 3

As quickly as it starts boiling you pour the parboiled rice cook for 20-30 minutes till the water gets dry then your rice is equipped.

<u>Fried Chicken and traditional jellof rice with locust beans</u>

Ingredients

100g of uncooked chicken

Sliced onions

5 cubes of Maggi

Spices

4 cups of red rice

½ cup vegetable oil

½ Palm oil

Blended pepper

3 tablespoonfuls of crayfish

2 tablespoonful of locust beans

Step 1

Wash 100g of uncooked chicken suitable and put it in a pot add 1 cups of water, add slice onion little quantity, add 1 Maggi and thyme and parboil for 15 minutes

Step 2

After the chicken is cooked you get an easy frypan, add ½ cup of vegetable oil and heat, then you put the hen barring the water and enable it to fry for 3 minutes and then your fried chicken is ready.

Step 3

For the rice - you get a easy pot pour 4 cups of rice add water and put it on fireplace and enable to parboil for 5 minutes thereafter you do away with the pot from furnace wash the rice with filter, then you put the empty pot on furnace and add ½ cup of Palm oil, add blended onion and pepper, stir and allow to fry for two minutes add 3 tablespoon of crayfish you stir and add two cups of water, add three Maggie cubes and Locust beans cowl the pot and allow to boil so that the elements can combine top

Step 4

As quickly as it starts off, you add salt to taste, thereafter you pour your rice in the pot, cowl it and allow it to cook and for the water to dry as soon as the water gets dried your standard rice with Locust beans is ready.

<u>Egusi soup with locust beans</u>

Ingredients

2 cups of grounded egusi

Stock fish

Blended onions and pepper

2 tablespoonful of locust beans

Bitter leaf

Uziza seed

Seasoning of your choice

Palm oil

Salt

Step 1

Great your pepper, onions and set aside, soaked your stock fish in hot water for 5 minutes

Step 2

Wash your bitter leaf and keep aside, blend the locust beans, uziza seed, and your seasoning in one place and set aside

Step 3

In a pot, add Palm oil and fry, add your blended pepper and onion,stir fry for 3 minutes,add your inventory fish and stir for a while

Step 4

In a plate, put your egusi and add a little water stir, and put it in your pot and stir fry for 3 minutes then add your seasoning, uziza seed and locust beans stir once more for two minutes and add your little water then cowl your pot for some minutes

Step 5

After some mins open your put and add your washed bitter leaf a little by little and stir very well and cowl the pot for a couple of minutes

Step 6

Your soup is ready to serve.

## Method of processing and preparing of locust beans for cooking

<u>Processing Stages</u>

The identified processing degrees concerned in processing of African locust bean can be introduced as follows:

Stage 1

African Locust Bean Seeds

stage 2

Boil in Water for 12 to 24 hours

stage 3

Cooling

stage 4

De-hulling by pressing with fingers or foot

Stage 5

Washing

stage 6

Discard/Separation of seed coats and selection

Stage 7

Re-boiling for every other 1½-2 hours in water with or besides native rock salt

Stage 8

Undergo fermentation

Stage 9

Production of gentle locust bean (salting in water and the use of salted water in molding is for soft ones into balls)

Stage 10

Production of dry locust bean (salting of water and the use of salted water in molding is for soft ones into balls)

## Processing and preparing of locust beans flowchart

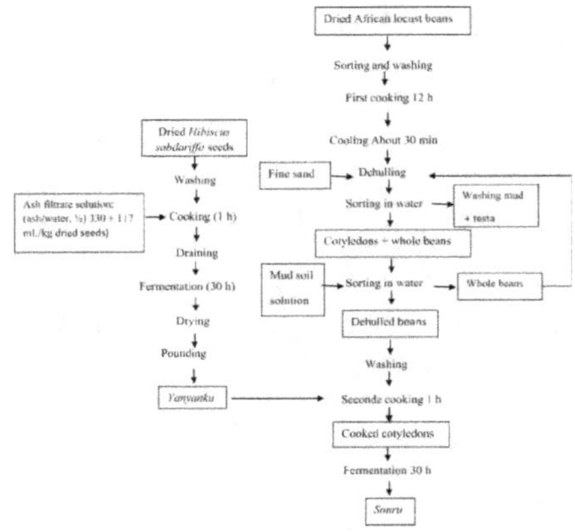


## Traditional ways of preserving/sun-drying locust beans

Wash and clean the beans

Spread out the locust beans

Turn it regularly

Cover the beans at night

Check for dryness

Store the dried beans for future use

**The versatility of locust beans spiritually and ritual ceremonies**

<u>Bringing precise luck</u>

Locust beans are believed to deliver excellent success to those who use them. They are regularly used in rituals and ceremonies to entice prosperity and abundance. it is said that by carrying locust beans or using them in rituals on can ta into the effective electricity of the universe and occur properly fortune

<u>Warding off evil spirits</u>

Locust beans are frequently used in usual African medicine to ward off evil spirits. It is believed that the robust smell of the beans is repulsive to evil spirits, and that by using them, one can create a protecting barrier towards poor energy.

Protecting against bad energy

In addition to warding off evil spirits, locust beans are additionally believed to guard towards bad energy. This includes bad thoughts, feelings and intentions from others. It is said that by way of carrying locust beans or using them in rituals, one can create guard of wonderful power that repels negativity